AF510826

Feel Better Now...Meditation

Feel Better Now... Meditation

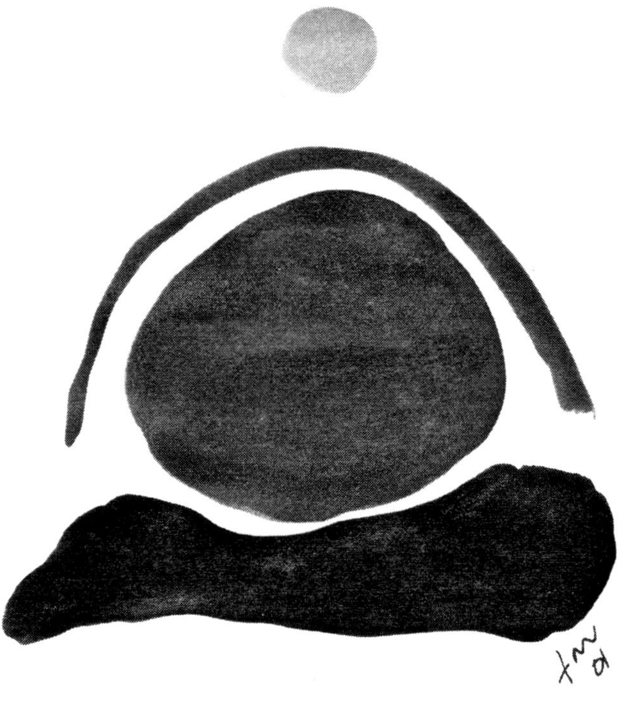

for Stress Reduction & Relaxation

Gary Halperin

Avid Reader Press

Avid Reader Press, Reno NV 89502
www.AvidReaderPress.com
© 2003 by Gary Halperin

All rights reserved. Published 2003. No part of this book shall be reproduced, stored in a retrieval system, or transmitted by any means, electronic, mechanical, photocopying, recording, or otherwise, without express written permission from the publisher. Printed in the United States of America.

07 06 05 04 03 5 4 3 2 1

Library of Congress Cataloging-in-Publication Data

Halperin, Gary
Feel better now. . . meditation: for stress reduction and relaxation

p. cm.
Includes index.
LCCN 2002113739
ISBN 0-9700150-2-X
1. Meditation. I. Title.
BF637.M4H35 2003 158.1'2
QBI03-200036

For Educational Purposes Only

This publication is designed to provide information in regard to the subject matter covered. While a great deal of care has been taken to provide accurate and current information, neither the author, publisher, its editor nor staff assume responsibility for the accuracy of the data contained herein.

This publication is sold with the understanding that the publisher is not engaged in rendering medical services or any other professional service. If medical advice or other expert assistence is required, the services of a competent professional should be sought. This publication is sold for educational purposes only. No liability is assumed for damages resulting from the use of the information contained herein.

This book is dedicated to my wife Rose *Anne—*
my playmate, my love, and my eternal inspiration.

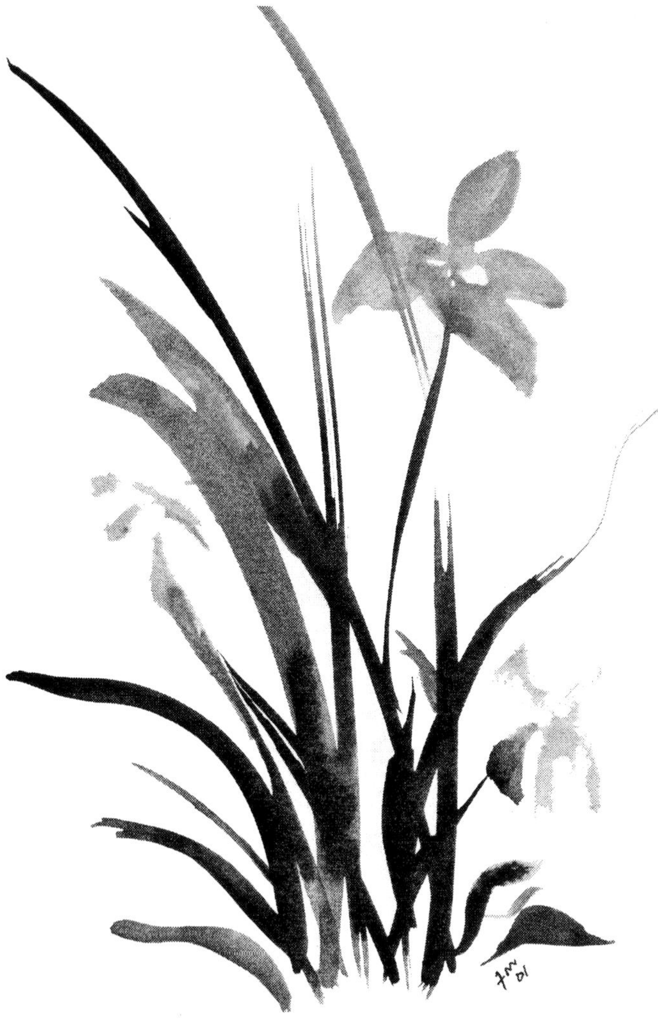

Preface

I was born into a family of high achievers. Until I was twenty-four, I never questioned in my mind that my life's purpose was to be outwardly successful. So I succeeded.

In high school, I was the valedictorian, captain of the basketball team, and voted by my peers as "most likely to succeed." I graduated from Amherst College in Massachusetts with a degree in political science and, in 1990, entered the United States Peace Corps in the Dominican Republic.

When I returned, I wondered what to do next. For the first time in my life, I felt like I needed to get away from my family and friends and spend some time alone thinking about what I wanted to do and who I wanted to be.

Without knowing at all what I was getting into, I went for a two week retreat to the Kripalu Center for Yoga and Health in Lenox, Massachusetts. I had never done yoga before. In fact, I did not even know what yoga was or what a yoga class looked like. Yet somehow I had a felt sense that I had come to the right place to experience and learn something new and valuable.

At Kripalu I was exposed for the first time to "Eastern thought." I began a journey inward. I questioned if the purpose of my life was to be outwardly successful. I learned that there was another way to approach and think about life that was not based on worldly success but on cultivating compassion, balance, peace, acceptance, presence, and non-judgmental awareness within myself.

A year later I joined the staff at the Kripalu Center where I lived and worked for three years. At that time, besides being a guest retreat center, Kripalu was a residential community (an ashram) of 300 people dedicated to living a spiritual life. We practiced yoga, meditation, conscious communication and selfless service together each day. Before leaving the ashram, I was certified as a Kripalu Yoga Teacher and Holistic Lifestyle Teacher.

From 1994 to 1996 I taught yoga and meditation at Kripalu, at a retreat center in San Jose, Costa Rica and privately in Northampton, Massachusetts. In the fall of 1996, I took a position as Spa Programs Director and Yoga and Meditation Instructor at Coolfont Resort in Berkeley Springs, West Virginia.

Soon after my arrival at Coolfont, the mayor of a major east coast city came to the resort with his fifty top administrators for a retreat. The group's retreat planner asked if there was someone on staff at Coolfont who could give them an hour-long session on meditation and spirituality, and he was referred to me. I took this opportunity to refine how I thought about and taught meditation. The workshop I planned and delivered was the genesis for this book.

⁂

This book explains what meditation is, how to meditate, the benefits of meditation, and answers frequently asked questions. It is not preachy or "new-agey" or affiliated with any religious or specific spiritual point of view. It is straightforward and to-the-point so that you can pick up and, in one or a few sittings, learn how and why to meditate. The frequently asked questions section is designed to answer questions that often come up when you begin to practice meditation.

This book is for anyone who wants to learn a method to relax, people who have never meditated and want to learn, and experienced meditators who want a new perspective on the practice. The central point is that meditation is about practicing focusing on process and not results—meditation is not about achieving or performing.

Many people, even people who meditate, are under the mistaken impression that to meditate means to keep the mind focused on something or "to clear the mind."

In fact, the benefits of meditation come from the mind-set that you are not trying to achieve or accomplish anything when you are practicing. This book explains this point of view and makes clear the relationship between how to meditate and the benefits that come from meditating.

⁂ ⁂ ⁂

I taught meditation workshops and gave private meditation instruction at Coolfont Resort for three years. Subsequently, I taught meditation at the Grandover Resort in Greensboro, North Carolina where I was the Spa Director. Now I teach meditation and yoga privately to individuals and groups in Sarasota, Florida.

I have noticed a rapidly growing interest in this topic. Many people want to learn to relax or slow down or broaden their perspective on life and have heard that meditation may be a good way to do these things.

Several of my students have asked me to suggest a book that is short and to-the-point and that covers what I teach in my Meditation for Stress Reduction workshops. I know of no book that meets these criteria. So I have written one.

⁂ ⁂ ⁂

My hope is that this book will assist you in some way on your inward journey.

Gary Halperin
Sarasota, Florida
2003

In appreciation for their assistance in the creation of this book, I thank Joe Young, Ina Young, Amy Summers-Hayes, William Schief, Kimberly Rossi, Norman Rosenthal, Carol Pitchersky, Fjola Petursdottir, Neal Owens, Daniel Martin, the Malina family, Ken McRae, the McCabe family, Matthew London, Elena Lipkowski, Robert Levine, Bruce Leblang, Kathleen Knipp, Jean Hurley, Jane Henley, Sachin Hazen, Peter Hartmann, Laura Hartmann, Carolyn Hartmann, Morton Halperin, Mark Halperin, David Halperin, David Goldstein, Beverly Goldberg, Scott Garber, Barry Friedman, Hannah Cole, Joel Caplan, Sharon Brash, James Bellevue, Karen Avrich, Martha Ashelman, the founders and staff of the Kripalu Center for Yoga and Health, and my grandparents.

And I wish to thank everyone else who has assisted me on my journey. May God bless all of you.

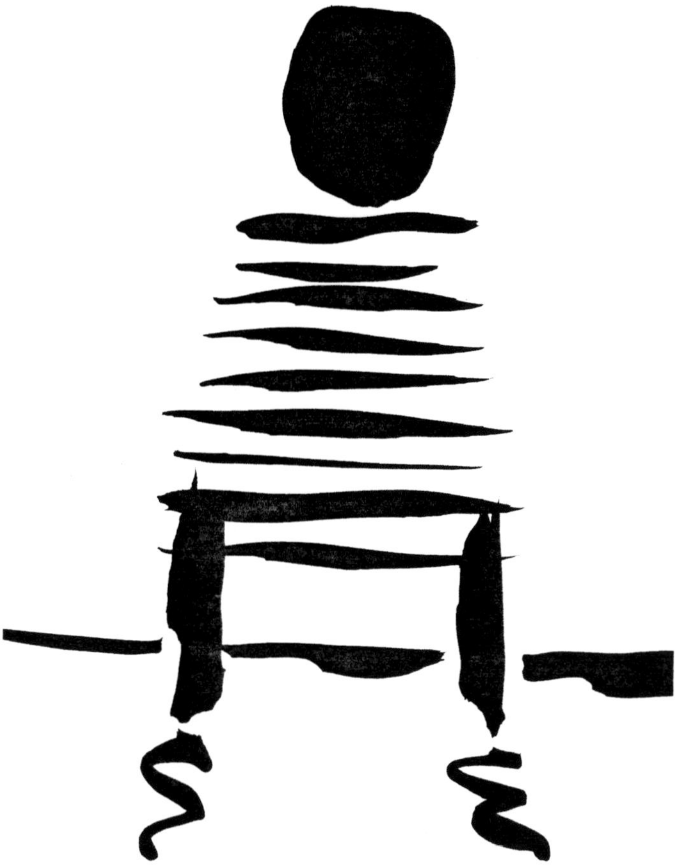

Introduction

A man meets his friend on the street.

"How are you doing, Harry? Hey, has your son found a job yet?"

"No, he is still looking. He has been doing a lot of meditation."

"Oh yeah, I've heard that word a lot lately. What exactly is meditation?"

"I don't know. But it's better than just sitting around doing nothing."

Meditation is better than just sitting around doing nothing. And paradoxically, it is just sitting and doing nothing.

⁂ ⁂ ⁂

There are many different ways of talking about and practicing meditation. This book explains the philosophy and method I have developed, taking the best of what I have learned from others. I have been trained in Kripalu Meditation and Siddha Samahdi Yoga Meditation, and I have studied other methods including Transcendental Meditation and Vipassana Meditation.

If meditation were the Atlantic Ocean, this book would be like sticking a teaspoon into the ocean, drawing it out and saying "What is in this spoon is the Atlantic Ocean." It is and it isn't. This book will contain many of the elements and the essence of meditation. It is not the whole ocean; it is not everything one could say about meditation.

⁂ ⁂ ⁂

※ ※ ※

The first part of this book discusses what meditation is, how to meditate, and the benefits it offers. The benefits of meditation include relaxation, acceptance, stress-reduction, improved decision making, and an increased appreciation for life. Once you have tried meditation, you may have many questions.

The second part of this book will give answers to questions frequently asked by beginners to meditation.

※ ※ ※

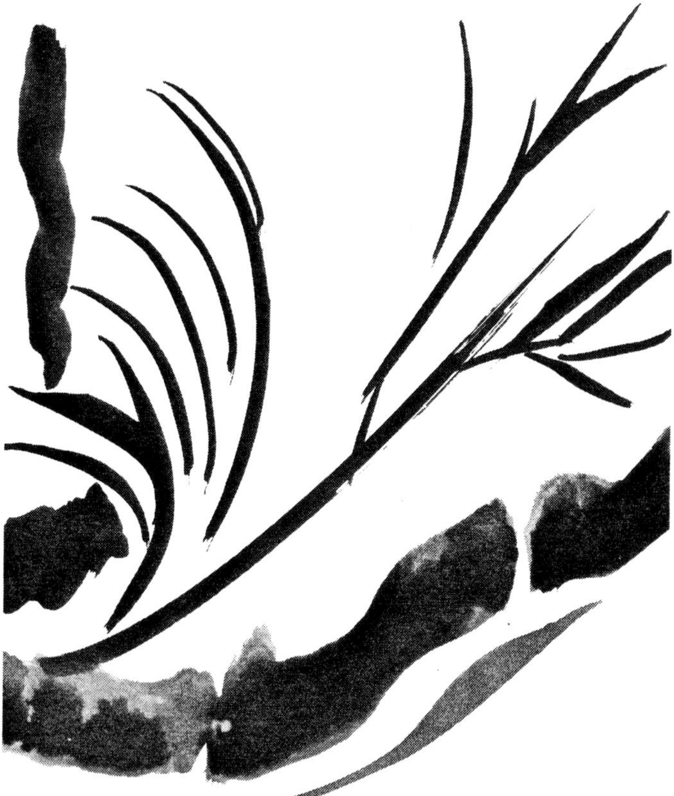

What is Meditation?

A way to begin talking about what meditation is, is to talk about what it is not—to make some distinctions.

If you are thinking about a problem or a person over and over again with associated feelings of stress and anxiety, that is not meditation. You could call that worry or obsession. That may be something that you cannot stop doing, but it is certainly not meditation.

If you are thinking about a problem strategically or

intellectually or having what appears to you to be great insights about your life, that is not meditating. You could call that contemplation. That may be something you want to do, but it is not meditation.

If you are sitting or lying down and just letting your mind go wherever it wants to go without using any technique, that is not meditation. You could call that resting or relaxing. That also may be something you want to do, but it is not meditation.

So this begs the question, "what is meditation?" Meditation is the practice of noticing when the mind wanders. Or, more precisely, meditation is the practice of being aware of when the mind moves off a chosen point of focus.

The chosen point of focus can be called the anchor—the anchor of the meditation. Often the name for a type of meditation will come from the name of the anchor. You might have a breath meditation or a sound meditation or a mantra meditation, these are all anchors. Or the anchor could be the sensations you feel in your body, what you see with your eyes closed, or a prayer or affirmation.

What makes these things effective anchors is that they are happening all the time and if something is happening all the time, it is happening now. Anchors are all present moment experiences.

The anchor can be your breath right now, what you feel in your body right now, the sounds you are hearing right now, the sensations you feel in your body right now, or if the anchor is a mantra or prayer or affirmation, it is what you are saying right now.

Meditation is the practice of being aware of when the mind moves off a chosen point of focus. Another way of saying it is that meditation is the practice of being aware of when the mind moves out of the present moment. When you notice that the mind is off your anchor—out of the present—you gently come back to the present by coming back to the anchor.

A way to think about the anchor is to use the "puppy analogy." When you buy a puppy and decide to teach it to sit, you may say to the dog a thousand times "sit, sit, sit," but the dog won't sit. The way you make the dog sit the first time is to place your hand on its backside and gently press it down as you say "sit."

That is analogous to what you are doing with the anchor and the mind. You are using the anchor to sit the mind down in the present moment. Imagine gently pressing the mind down so that it is sitting in the present.

The nature of the puppy, however, is to roam around. So, too, is the nature of the mind. You can sit the mind down in the present, but very soon thereafter it will get up and move around just as the puppy does.

After you sit the dog down, you could turn to a friend and say, "Look, I got my dog to sit." However, as soon as you turn, the dog will probably get up and move around. You know right away when the puppy gets up and moves around. The difference between a dog sitting and a dog moving around is easy to notice. Noticing when the mind moves is more difficult for two reasons.

First, you need to use your mind to notice your mind. And that is a skill you develop when you meditate—the skill of using your mind to notice your mind.

Second, you need to notice where the mind has gone. If you let a dog loose in a room, you can see where it is. The area is limited, bounded, and finite. Where the mind can go is unlimited, unbounded, and infinite. This area includes everything you have ever experienced, everything you have taken in consciously and unconsciously, everything you want to happen in the future, and everything you are afraid could happen in the future. The range of places the mind can go is vast and to notice your mind in so huge a territory is not easy. It is a skill. And it is a skill you develop when you meditate—the skill of noticing where the mind is. We will explore why it is useful to notice the mind when we discuss the benefits of meditation. For now, all we are talking about is technique.

Again, meditation is the practice of being aware of when the mind moves off a chosen point of focus. The chosen point of focus is called the anchor. These statements are important as definitions. The next thing I am going to tell you is the key to understanding meditation.

How long you stay on your anchor in between wanderings of the mind and overall during the course of the meditation is not important. You are still going to get the benefits of meditation simply by having an anchor and having an intention to come back to the anchor when you notice that you are off it.

To repeat, how long you stay on your anchor in between wanderings of the mind and overall during the course of the meditation is not important. You are still going to get the benefits of meditation simply by having an anchor and having an intention to come back to the anchor when you notice that you are off it.

For many people this is a hard concept to take in. In my workshops I will state the above idea, people will nod their heads, and many could probably even repeat it back to me. Then we meditate, and I ask them what happened.

Some say "Well, I got really frustrated, I couldn't stay on my anchor." Others will say after meditating, "That was hard." "What was hard?" I ask. "It was hard to stay on my anchor." I agree that staying on the anchor is hard. Luckily, that is not what we are trying to do. The benefits of meditation do not, in any way, require you to stay on your anchor.

I remind my students that meditation is not about

staying on the anchor, and it is not even about quickly noticing when you are off the anchor. Meditation is simply about choosing an anchor and making an intention to come back to the anchor when you notice that you are off it—that is, when you happen to notice that you are off it.

When you meditate, you are training yourself not to worry about the mind being off the anchor. When you are meditating, you are not trying to do anything or be attached to any particular outcome. Your goal is to simply be involved in the process.

Again, for many people this is a hard concept to take in. With most activities first you learn how to do them. Then your next questions are "How do I get good at this?" "How do I achieve at this?" "How do I know that I am doing this right?"

Meditation is a different type of activity. It is not about achieving, it is about non-achieving. It is not about doing, it is about non-doing. It is not about results, it is about process. Meditation is not a performance.

When you meditate you bring yourself to a safe

comfortable environment. You choose an anchor and make an intention to come back to the anchor when you notice that you are off it. That is it. That is the whole process. By focusing on the process and not results you will get many of the benefits of meditation.

※ ※ ※

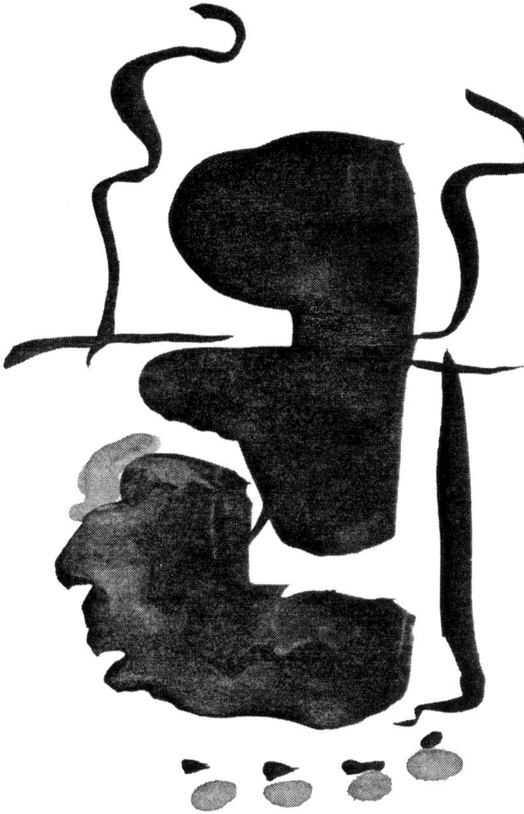

How to Meditate

To practice meditation, bring yourself to a quiet and safe environment where you will feel comfortable spending some time with your eyes closed and your focus inward. You could be in a nice place in your home, or outside in a park, or even at your desk at work. If possible and convenient, wear loose fitting, comfortable clothing and take off your shoes.

Do your best to limit the possibility of external distractions: turn off the telephone ringer, tell others at home or at work you wish not to be disturbed for a period of time, and close the windows if there may be unpleasant sounds from the outside.

Set an alarm or timer to go off at the time you wish to end your meditation. Beginners can start with five or ten minute sessions and increase the meditation time as they become more experienced and if they so choose.

Sit in a comfortable position on the floor or on a chair or sofa. Close your eyes and choose a point of focus (or anchor) on which to meditate. Make an intention to bring your attention back to your anchor whenever you become aware that your mind has wandered. Put your mind's attention on the anchor. Each time you notice that your mind has moved off your chosen anchor, gently remind yourself to focus back on your anchor.

※ ※ ※

Do not worry about how long you actually stay on the point of focus in between wanderings of the mind. The time will vary for everyone for each meditation. As long as you have an anchor and an intention to keep returning to it whenever you are aware that your mind has wandered off it, you are meditating correctly. When the timer or alarm sounds, end your meditation session by gently opening your eyes.

⁂ ⁂ ⁂

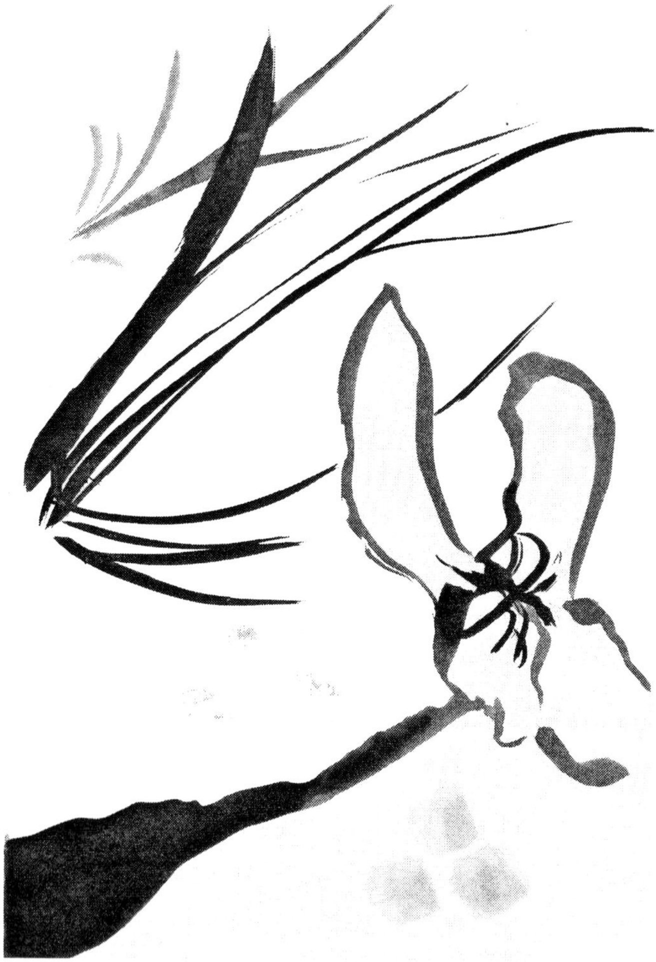

Benefits of Meditation

We have talked about what meditation is—the practice of being aware of when the mind moves off a chosen point of focus. We have also talked about how to meditate: set yourself up in the proper environment, close your eyes, choose an anchor, and make an intention to come back to the anchor, when you notice that you are off it.

Now the question is why you would want to do this. What are the benefits of meditation? The benefits of meditation include relaxation, acceptance, stress-reduction, improved decision making, and an increased appreciation for life.

Relaxation

Often when people meditate they feel relaxed. Having an internal experience with a "non-doing attitude," without striving or struggling or trying, tends to create relaxation. All the pressure is off. The meditator is simply focused on the process.

A feeling of relaxation also may be created by the environment in which you have chosen to meditate. In fact, spending quiet time in a safe, comfortable environment with your eyes closed can induce relaxation even if you are not meditating. So one obvious possible benefit of meditation is to create relaxation during the practice that may last some time after the practice.

Acceptance

Meditation is often relaxing; however, you won't always feel relaxed while you meditate. Sometimes you might feel anxious, sometimes you might feel afraid, or sometimes you might feel bored. Sitting down and focusing on an anchor can be boring.

Part of what you are learning when you meditate is acceptance: being with whatever is, without trying to change it or fix it. This is a second benefit of meditation. Sitting and experiencing some negative feelings or emotions, if that is what is happening, will not kill you. So for once in your life, if you are feeling uncomfortable, you are not going to pick up the phone or talk to anyone or turn on the TV. You are not going to read a newspaper or eat or even move. You are just going to sit there without trying to change your emotions or feelings. You are going to let whatever happens, happen.

What you will notice often happens is that the feelings or emotions change. So you might start out feeling anxious or bored and, then you might notice that you are feeling relaxed. Then you might feel anxious again. The idea is to be with whatever happens, without trying to change it.

So for ten or fifteen minutes—however long you decide to meditate—you are just going to let whatever happens happen. It is not for the rest of your life. Just for a set period you are going to experiment with not trying to fix what may appear to feel uncomfortable.

Part of what you are learning when you meditate is that your feelings or emotions will often change without you doing anything. You may plan to feel relaxed when meditating, however that may not be the case, so you just stay with the process and let the results take care of themselves. In this way, you develop the quality of acceptance. We will return briefly to this discussion of how the practice of meditation can lead to the quality of acceptance after you have completed your first meditation using the technique explained in this book.

Stress-Reduction

We have discussed two benefits of meditation: relaxation and acceptance. A third benefit is stress reduction. Let's look at how meditation can help reduce stress in your daily life.

When you meditate, you focus on process and not results. Whenever you focus on the process of what you are doing and not the result, you are reducing stress. This is because you are focusing on what you largely can control, what you are presently doing, instead of what you can largely not control, how something may come out, or what others may say about what you have done.

So when you meditate, you sit down in a safe comfortable quiet environment, you bring an anchor to mind and make an intention to come back to the anchor when you notice that you are off it. You are not trying to achieve anything. You are not performing. You are not trying to stay on your anchor. And you are not trying to notice quickly when you are off it. You simply are involved with the process of gently coming back when you happen to notice you are off your anchor.

This process is all contained within your head. No one else knows what you are thinking about and no one else cares. Meditation is your own private, personal experience. In that environment, can you practice giving yourself a break? Can you practice not worrying about how long you are on or off your anchor?

For some people, this is very difficult to grasp. Even knowing the ground rules, some will start to meditate, notice they are off their anchors, and then start having thoughts such as "Oh, my god, I am off my anchor. I don't know how long I have been off my anchor. I am no good at this. I don't know how to meditate."

Having these types of thoughts are normal. When you meditate, you practice noticing these thoughts and then coming back to your anchor. You stay with the process as best as you can and do not worry about straying away from the process. With each moment, you have another chance to come back to your anchor.

By keeping in mind that you are not trying to achieve anything, you are not performing, and you are simply involved in the process, you make the meditation practice itself a no-stress or very low stress experience. In this way, you are taking all the pressure off of yourself. Again, whenever you allow yourself to be involved with process and not results, you reduce the stress in whatever you are doing.

This philosophy behind meditation can be taken out into the world and applied where you choose. For example, let's say you are cooking a meal for friends or colleagues or family members or a date. It is a meal that is important to you.

While you are cooking, you may start thinking "I am not sure if that person likes this type of food" or "these foods don't really go together" or "this is not fancy enough for that person" or "it's not all going to come out at the right time." These thoughts can be called negative predictions about the future.

Having these thoughts is very natural and normal. When you practice meditation, focusing on process and not results, you are more likely to notice you are having these negative thoughts when you are cooking and then come back to the process itself—come back to the process of cooking. You could then focus on cutting vegetables or filling pots with water or taking things out of the refrigerator or details of the recipe. And if that process seems too tedious, you could be listening to music playing in your kitchen. When you notice that you not listening to music, when you are having negative predictions about the future, you come back to the music. Applying the meditation principle of focusing on the moment, of focusing on process and not results, can be called mindfulness.

When you do this, you may get better results even though you are not focusing on results. When you are mindful of what you are doing in the moment and not on what may or may not happen later or on what people may or may not say later, you may end up doing a better job.

But I am not telling you that this is a good way to get positive results. I am telling you that the practice of mindfulness will bring down the stress in whatever you are doing, and you may also get better results.

Let's look at another example of how you can use meditation practice to reduce stress. Let's say you get into your car after work one day and start to drive home and you notice that there is more traffic than usual. You may have the thought: "This is going to make me fifteen minutes later than normal," and then automatically get into a result-oriented action. You might start driving faster or switching lanes or cutting off other drivers or getting angry with other drivers all because you believe, without thinking about it, that the result of getting home at the regular time is very important.

When you practice meditation and practice focusing on process and not results, you are more likely to ask yourself the questions, "Does the result really matter in this case? Is there someone even waiting for me? And if there is, Would it be okay if I were fifteen minutes late?"

In this case you may decide that the result is not crucial, and you can come back to the process—the process of driving the car. You can focus on what you see out the window, what you are feeling in your body, what sounds you are hearing, your breathing, or if that

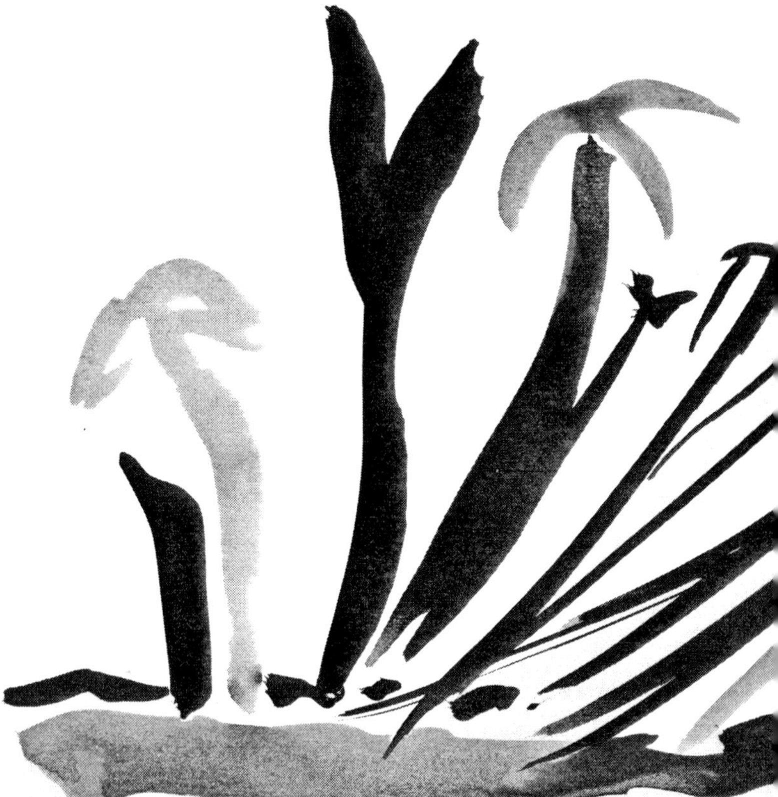

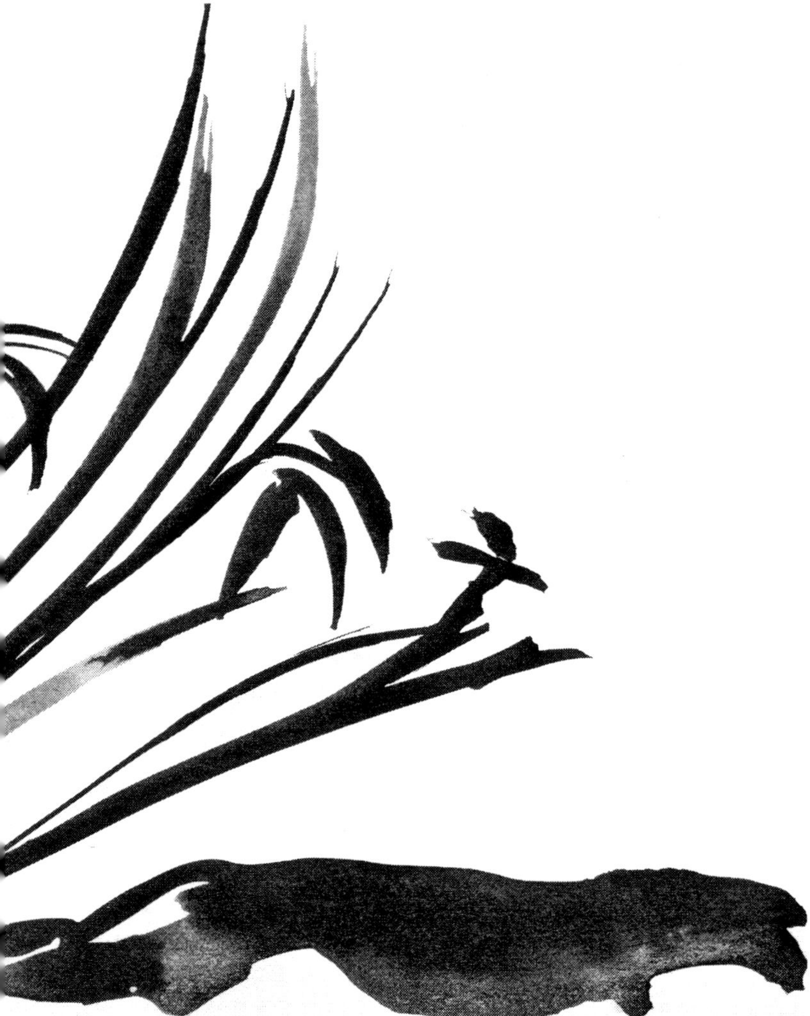

seems too tedious, you could turn on the radio and focus on what is on the radio. When you notice that you are having thoughts about results or getting into actions related to results, you bring your mind back to the process—the process of driving.

In other cases, you might say that results are important to you. Perhaps you feel that your job demands results or your investments demand results. That is fine. Where results are important to you, go ahead and focus on results. But certainly there are some areas of your life where you can allow yourself to focus on process. The question then becomes where do you begin?

Well, you begin with the practice of formal meditation. In a safe, comfortable, peaceful environment, you choose an anchor and then make an intention to come back to the anchor when you notice that you are off it. You are not trying to achieve anything. You are simply involved with the process.

And again, you decide how you want to apply this practice of meditation in your life. So as a final example, let's say you are swimming in a pool. You can either be focused on thoughts such as "Am I going as fast as I normally go? Am I burning enough calories? Is chlorine getting in my hair? Am I going to be late for my next appointment?" or you can notice that you are having those thoughts and then come back to the process of swimming itself. You might notice the feeling of your arms and legs moving in the water, or focus on your breathing as your face turns from surface to water and back. Again, whenever you do this, if you allow yourself to focus on process and not results, you are going reduce the stress in whatever you are doing.

Improved Decision Making

We have discussed three benefits of meditation: relaxation, acceptance, and stress-reduction. Another benefit of meditation is improved decision making. This benefit is related to the ideas expressed in the best selling book *Emotional Intelligence* by Daniel Goleman. Goleman discusses how it is possible to raise one's "emotional intelligence" and how this intelligence can lead to a more satisfying and productive life. I will devote more space to this benefit than the others as I have found that many of my students find it the most relevant to their daily life.

Improving one's ability to make decisions is a way to increase one's "emotional intelligence" and this is possible through meditation. I am referring to a specific kind of decision that comes up when the body is under stress—when you are having what is called a "flight or fight response."

As human beings we are all wired in emergencies to be able to act without thinking. For example, if your baby falls in the swimming pool, you will jump in the pool and try to save the baby without thinking. That action is an automatic response to an emergency situation, and it is appropriate and useful. Of course people who were not wired to protect their progeny died out a long time ago.

A difficulty occurs when the mind tells you that something is an emergency situation and leads you to an automatic response in a situation that is not really an immediate emergency. In its effort to protect you, the mind is constantly looking for danger and emergencies. And in response to what it perceives, the mind will tell you that this is happening and it could lead to something else, which could lead to something else, so you'd better take some immediate action.

In your body you will feel like you are experiencing an emergency that demands an automatic response. You will have what Dr. Herbert Benson, in his book *The Relaxation Response,* called the "stress response." The same bodily reactions will happen to some degree as when the baby falls in the pool. Among other reactions, your blood pressure goes up, your heart starts beating faster, and you start to secrete certain hormones. You feel like you are or someone else is about to die, and you had better act quickly.

When you practice meditation, you develop the skill of using the mind to notice the mind. You develop the skill of noticing the mind wandering. Your meditation practice can give you skills so that when you get into a stressful situation and the mind is jumping from thought to thought to thought, which might lead you to an action, you are more likely to notice these mind jumps. Then you can come back to what really is happening or just happened and decide what you want to do instead of having an automatic response to a situation that may not demand an automatic response.

Perhaps an example will make this clearer. Let's say you are at work, and you pass your supervisor in the hall, and her expression seems to indicate that she is angry or unhappy. You may have the thoughts, "she is angry, she is angry at me, I've done something wrong."

And then you may think, "I might lose my job. If I lose my job, I can't make my house payments, and I can't make my car payments, and my spouse may leave me." And then you may return to your office and think, "Well, you know what, I never really liked this job anyway, and I don't like her." And then you may think, "Well, she asked me to do that memo three weeks ago, I haven't done it, I think I will do that now."

Activity in the mind in this type of situation can be very fast and furious: you may feel like you are dying, you may feel as if your baby is in the swimming pool. When you practice meditation and develop the skill of using the mind to notice the mind, you are more likely, in this type of situation, to notice the mind jumping. You can then stop the process at any point, come back to what really happened, or is happening, and decide what you want to do instead of automatically responding to a situation that does not demand an automatic response.

So you can pass your supervisor in the hall and notice her expression and have the thought, "She's angry, she's angry at me." Stop the process there. Or when you think, "I am going to lose my job and, then I can't make my car payments," stop the process there. Wherever you can, notice the mind jumping, stop the process, and then come back to what really happened.

So what really happened? You passed your supervisor in the hall and she looked unhappy. You can now think, "Maybe she is not unhappy, maybe she has indigestion, or maybe I am just misinterpreting the look. . . Or, maybe she is unhappy, but she certainly may not be unhappy with me. What do I choose to do about it?"

Maybe you would return to your office and call her and say, "I passed you in the hall, you looked unhappy to me. Am I imagining there is something wrong? Is there something I can do for you?" Or maybe you don't have that type of relationship with your boss, so instead you might get back to your office and think, "She looked unhappy. I don't know, maybe she is unhappy with me, maybe she is not. She did ask me to do that memo three weeks ago, so I will cover my bases and do that now."

Thus you might end up with the same action anyway. But you get there by looking at what really happened, from a place of slowing down, from a place of consciousness, instead of having an automatic response to a situation that does not demand an automatic response.

The practice of meditation is akin to digging the well before the house is on fire. You do not formally practice meditation when you are feeling under intense stress. You choose to meditate—dig your well—when you are feeling relatively stable and not under attack from the world—when the house is not on fire. Then you go out into the world and when potentially stressful things happen, you have built up a reservoir of skill and practice to draw upon. Now, when it feels like your house is on fire, you are more likely to notice the mind jumping and come back to what is really happening then make a decision about what you want to do.

Let's look at another, somewhat lighter, example where the skill developed in meditation of using the mind to notice the mind could be useful. Let's say you are at a party and go through a buffet line. Then you sit down, and you eat the lobster soufflé you have selected. It is wonderful, it tastes great. What do you immediately think?

"Is there more? Is it going to run out? Should I get up and get more now?" Your heart may be pounding as a result of this dilemma. The possibility of not having more soufflé might feel like death itself is upon you. And you may move into immediate action.

Instead of enjoying the food you have, you may get up and look to see if there is any lobster left. Then you may scan the room and make an estimate of how many people may want the wonderful lobster soufflé. You may react by rushing back to the serving tables.

When you practice the skill of using the mind to

notice the mind through the formal practice of meditation, you might notice the mind jumping from "this is great" to "can I get more?" to "will it run out?" and then bring yourself back to the present and ask yourself what is happening.

You tasted the lobster soufflé, and it is really good. Now you are worrying about getting more. Maybe you will decide to think, "I might not get more, but right now I am not even enjoying what I already have. So instead of jumping up and running back to the buffet and maybe knocking into someone and embarrassing myself in the process, I am just going to enjoy the food I already have."

Increased Reverence or Appreciation for Life

We have covered four benefits of meditation—relaxation, acceptance, stress reduction and improved decision making. Now we will discuss a final benefit of meditation which is increased reverence for life, or you could call it increased appreciation for life.

This is really a very simple point. When you meditate, you practice slowing down and noticing more. Everything that you notice goes in the category of "I may appreciate this." Everything that you do not notice goes in the category of things you have no way to appreciate.

Close your eyes for about thirty seconds and notice what you hear. Right now. Close your eyes and just listen.

You probably heard some sounds that you were not aware of before. Where were those sounds before that short meditation? Where are they now? They are still happening, but you may be missing them. You might think, "Big deal. I am missing some sounds." But that is not the only thing you are missing in life. When you go through life never practicing the skill of slowing down and noticing, you might be missing all sorts of things that you don't want to miss.

You might miss something a colleague says or does that might make you appreciate him more or like him more. You might miss something that your child or grandchild or niece or nephew says or does. You might miss a view that you would want to see. Everything that you don't even notice goes in the category of things there is no way to appreciate; everything you notice goes in the category of things you may appreciate.

At one of my workshops, someone once said that this explanation of how meditation can create the benefit of increased appreciation of life reminded her of the saying "stop and smell the roses." But I am not simply saying "stop and smell the roses." I am saying that here is a practical way of developing the skill of stopping and smelling the roses—of learning how to notice more.

Most people would say that they want to appreciate their life more or life in general more. But this appreciation is not something you learn in school. Meditation is a practical, free way to develop the skill of noticing more so you can appreciate more.

Imagine what you see out the window if you are driving in your car at 100 miles per hour. You don't see much. Life is a blur at 100 miles per hour. But if you slow down, you might notice more. At sixty miles per hour you might see mountains and trees, and at thirty miles per hour you might see a child by the side of the road or an animal by the side of the road. The slower you go, the more you are going to notice. So when you get down to ten and nine and eight miles per hour, you are going to see more and more and more.

Everything you notice goes in the category of things you might appreciate. Everything in the blur is lost forever.

※ ※ ※

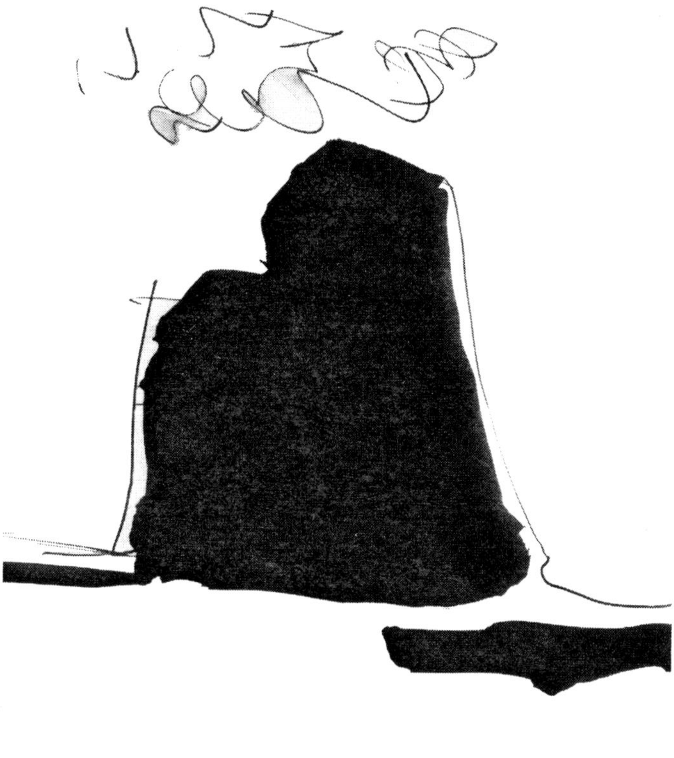

Meditation Practice and Anchors

You now have enough information to meditate and know why you would want to meditate. I would suggest you do a short meditation after completing this chapter. If you do not have the time, five to fifteen minutes, or inclination to meditate after reading this chapter, wait until you do before going on to read the next chapter.

If you have never meditated before, you may feel

uneasy, or even fearful, before you start. Doing anything for the first time can bring on some anxiety, and to some people meditation is a mysterious subject. The unknown tends to create unease. But remember, you are safe and will end up in the same place as where you started.

When you feel ready to meditate and have the time, find the most quiet and relaxed place you can and sit down (in a chair or on the floor). Choose an anchor. The anchor can be anything that is physically happening right now that you can experience with your eyes closed. Here are some suggestions.

You can focus on your breath. Some people focus on the breath coming in and out of their nostrils; some people focus on the breath coming in and out of the belly.

You can focus on the sounds you hear around you. You can listen to sounds and label and identify them: "That is a bird, that is a car passing by, that is my breath." Or you can listen to sounds the way a baby does—that is without identifying or labeling, just taking in the vibrations—what the sounds truly are. If you are using the latter method of just listening to sounds, and you notice that you are labeling or identifying sounds, you then come back to just listening.

You can focus on the sensations in your body. To do that, you bring your attention to your feet and scan up your body looking for any subtle or gross sensations and just noticing them. Come to the top of your head and then scan down, noting any sensations. When you notice that you are not doing a body scan, when the mind is somewhere else, you come back to the body scan.

You could focus on the internal, silent repetition of a mantra or affirmation or prayer. In this case, your anchor is what you are physically saying to yourself right now. A mantra is a sound or word or short phrase given to you by a meditation teacher or self-created. Some examples of mantras people use are "Om," "shalom," and "Om Namo Bhagavate Vasudevaya." Examples of affirmations you could use as your anchor are "I am at peace," "I am experiencing wellness," or, if you believe in God, "God loves me" or "God is with me." A prayer could be a brief, formal religious prayer or you can create one, such as "Oh, God, my heart is open, please come sit in my heart."

Your anchor can also be what you see with your eyes closed—not pictures but the lightness or darkness you might see. Some people can feel their heart beating and that could be an anchor. Some people feel an internal rocking sensation in their belly and that could be your anchor as well.

Once you have chosen an anchor, set a timer or alarm to go off when you wish the meditation to end. Choose a gentle sounding alarm—a bell or chime or soft classical music.

Sit up with your spine as straight as possible and close your eyes. Bring your anchor to mind. Then make an intention to come back to your anchor when you notice that you are off of it. Again, bring your anchor to mind and begin meditating. When the alarm sounds, take two deep breaths and then slowly open your eyes.

Meditate now. Remember the secret is not to stay on your anchor or even to notice quickly when you are off. The secret is not to care when you happen to notice your mind is somewhere else and then, with an attitude of total self-acceptance, gently come back to your anchor. The only way to do this wrong is to be judgmental about being off your anchor. The key is to cultivate non-judgmental self-awareness.

⁂ ⁂ ⁂

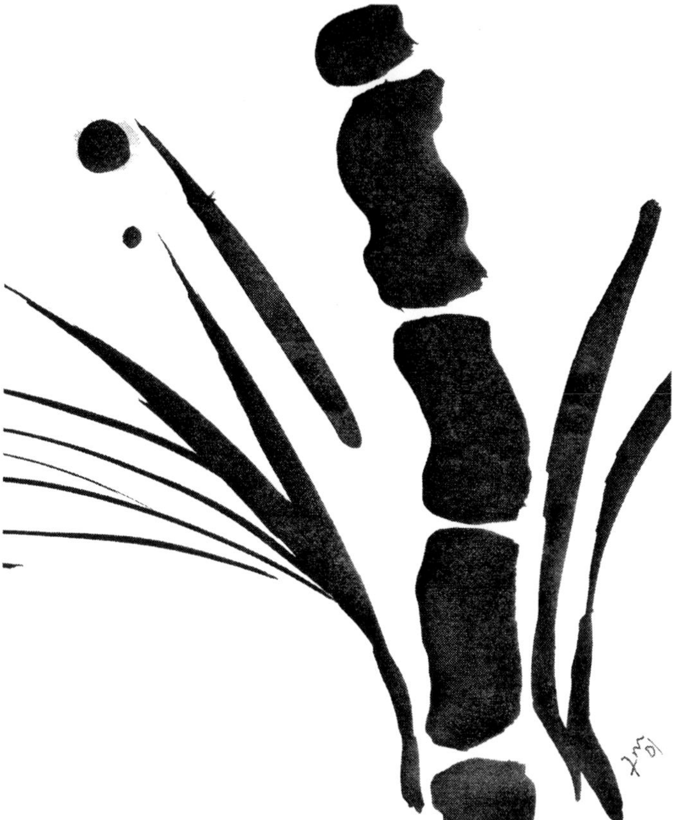

After Your First Meditation

Welcome back. I hope you had a pleasant inward journey. You might notice you feel more relaxed and have an enhanced sense of clarity. And you might not. Maybe your journey was not so pleasant. But note that you are still alive and that you have begun the process of developing some useful skills. As long as you had an anchor and came back to the anchor when you noticed when you were off it, you were meditating. You practiced focusing on process and not results, and you practiced using the mind to notice the mind.

During your meditation you might have felt distracted for some external or internal reason, maybe the phone rang or maybe there were loud noises or maybe you thought of something you have to do. There may have been distractions. Part of what you might discover when you meditate is that meditation is like life. When you meditate, other things may intervene; when you are living life, other things may intervene.

Some things might really bother you in life. Getting a phone call while you are having dinner can be annoying; getting a phone call while you are meditating can also be annoying. One of the things you are practicing when you meditate is letting go of things that are not of life or death consequence, that are not that important. You are learning to be not too serious. You are practicing acceptance. Maybe your meditation was interrupted by something. It is not a big deal. You are sitting, the process is all in your own mind. No one else is involved. Meditation is a personal experience in a private realm.

First of all, in this realm, give yourself a break.

When your mind wanders and you notice that wandering, do not chastise yourself for being off your anchor. Simply come back to the anchor, come back to the process. Also, give the world a break while you are meditating. If dogs are barking, wind is blowing, or the phone is ringing—as best as you can—recognize that this is not a big deal. Stay with the process of the meditation and the results, that is the benefits of meditation, will take care of themselves.

⁂ ⁂ ⁂

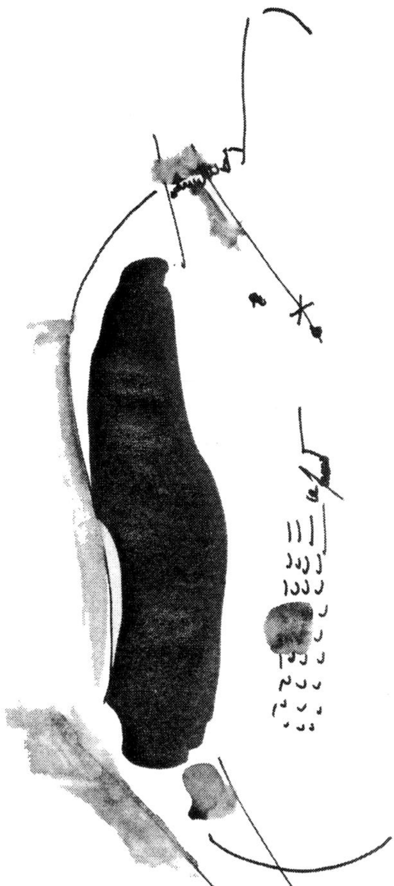

Review

Let's review what we have learned.

What is Meditation?

Meditation is the practice of noticing when the mind wanders or, more precisely, meditation is the practice of being aware of when the mind moves off a chosen point of focus. This point of focus is called the anchor.

Some anchors are breath, sounds, body sensations, prayer or affirmations, and what you see with your eyes closed.

⁂ ⁂ ⁂

How to Meditate

Sit comfortably in as quiet an environment as possible. Set a gentle alarm or timer to go off at the time you wish to end your meditation. Beginners can start with five or ten minute sessions and increase the time if they so choose and as they become more experienced. Close your eyes and choose a point of focus (or anchor) on which to meditate.

Make an intention to bring your attention back to your anchor whenever you become aware that your mind has wandered. Put your mind's attention on the anchor. Each time you notice that your mind has moved off your chosen anchor, gently remind yourself to focus back on your anchor.

Do not worry about how long you actually stay on the point of focus in between mind wanderings and overall. The time will vary for everyone in each meditation. As long as you have an anchor and an intention to keep returning to it whenever you are aware that your mind has wandered off it, you are meditating correctly.

When the timer or alarm sounds, end your meditation session by slowly opening your eyes.

⁂ ⁂ ⁂

Possible Benefits of Meditation

1. Relaxation
2. Acceptance
3. Stress reduction
4. Improved decision making
5. Increased appreciation or reverence for life

⁂ ⁂ ⁂

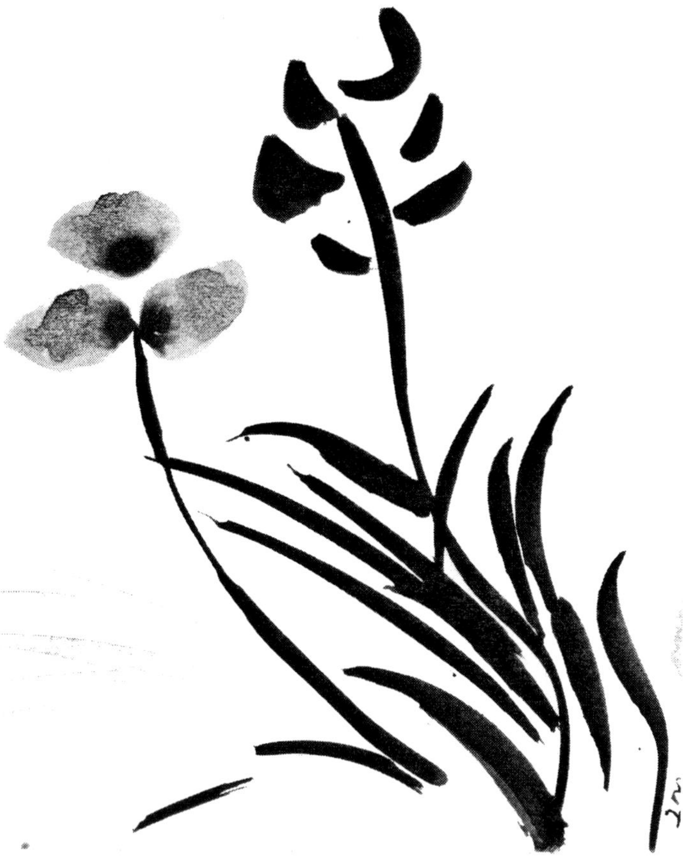

Frequent Questions

Is it okay to switch anchors during meditation?

There is a saying that "life is what happens when you make other plans." You can say the same thing about meditation. You might make a plan to have a certain anchor. Some things might intervene, and changing anchors during the meditation is okay. Some people just naturally fall into this practice.

You might decide to focus on your breath and then you begin to meditate, and you hear sounds like birds outside or a heater or air conditioner—some sounds that are keeping you from focusing on your breath. At that point switching your anchor to sounds is fine. As long as during the course of the meditation you are focusing on something that is happening now, you are going to get the benefits of meditation.

You might even make the intention at the beginning of the meditation to focus on whatever anchor happens to occur to you in any given moment. This can be called a roving meditation (perhaps the perfect meditation for the MTV generation that is used to quick cutting images and channel surfing). As long as you are not randomly switching anchors but are consciously deciding to switch, you are still going to get the benefits of meditation.

For example, you might begin by choosing to focus on your breath. You are on your breath, coming back to your breath, and then it occurs to you to focus on sounds. So you consciously choose to switch your anchor.

The anchor is ultimately just a substitute for the idea that "I am sitting here right now meditating." That concept can in fact be your anchor: "I am aware of myself in this room, physically here, meditating." When you are not aware of yourself in this room in this moment, when you notice your mind is somewhere else, come back to the realization that you are here now. The anchor is actually just a physical substitute for this thought.

※ ※ ※

When is the best time to meditate?

This is similar to the question of what is the best spiritual practice. The best spiritual practice is the one that you do. The best time to meditate is when you have time to meditate. If you have time in the morning, do it in the morning. If you have time in the middle of the day, do it then. If you have time in the evening or right before you go to bed, meditate then. Whenever you have the time to meditate, then practice.

If you have some flexibility, you can experiment with what times work best for you. Some people find that meditating in the morning gives them a feeling of clarity and peace that lasts during part or all of the day. Other people find that meditating at night helps them to relax and can even help them fall asleep.

※ ※ ※

How long should I meditate?

Start with five or ten or fifteen minutes and then increase over time if you so choose. I would recommend not to do more than thirty minutes on the basis of just the training in this book. If you want to meditate for more than thirty minutes, I suggest you go for some additional training in meditation.

⁂ ⁂ ⁂

How often should I meditate?

Like any other practice, to the extent that you meditate, to that extent you will realize the benefits of meditation. And there is no rush and no need to feel pressured to do more than you have time to do. One of my favorite expressions is "Patience is genius." You can apply that idea here. Meditation will not be a beneficial part of your life if it is another activity that you get stressed about if you feel that you are not doing it enough. A key point of meditation is to bring down your stress level. You will defeat that purpose if you worry about whether you meditate enough. The benefits of meditation are cumulative. You can take your time.

That said, if you have the time and inclination to meditate every day, then do it every day. And if you have time to do it twice a day, do it twice a day. And if you only have time to meditate once a week, then do it once a week. It is your own practice. You make the choice of how often you want to do it.

※ ※ ※

Is it okay to adjust my body while I am meditating?

Yes, especially if there is a pain or discomfort that is keeping you from your anchor. If this is happening, then adjust your position. Then focus your mind on your anchor.

※ ※ ※

Do I have to be sitting when I meditate? Can I be on my back?

You can definitely meditate lying on your back. The process is in your mind and can be practiced in any position. Some people find it useful to meditate on their back to help them fall asleep at night or if they wake up in the middle of the night and wish to resume sleeping.

⁕ ⁕ ⁕

If I am sitting, do I have to sit on the floor? Do I have to sit up straight?

You can sit on the floor, in a chair, or on a sofa. I recommend that you sit up as straight as you can while still being comfortable. If you need to lean back to be comfortable, then lean back as much as you need to.

There are two explanations that meditation teachers will give of why you should sit up as straight as possible. First, the straighter you are sitting, the more the body is in a learning and receptive mode. The mind and body are connected, so a receptive body will lead to a receptive mind. Your elementary school teacher had it right when he or she told you to sit up straight.

You can test this out right now with an experiment. Hunch your shoulders and learn forward. Notice how you feel. Now slowly straighten the spine and sit up straight. You can probably feel the difference immediately. When you sit up straight you are more likely to feel alert, awake, and ready to practice a new skill.

The second reason why a meditation teacher will tell you to sit up straight is more esoteric. Some people believe that the spine is a channel for energy in the body and that it is beneficial to move the energy up from the base of the spine to the head while you are in meditation. The straighter the spine is, the more easily the energy will rise.

⁂

In what environment should I meditate?

Choosing a quiet, safe, comfortable spot is best. You can be indoors or outdoors. Meditating in the same spot each day may help you feel relaxed and comfortable—perhaps sitting on your bed or in a chair, or sitting on the floor in a beautiful spot in your home or office.

Create a situation in which you are not likely to be disturbed. Turn off the telephone ringer. Tell others not to disturb you for a period of time. If possible and convenient, wear loose fitting, comfortable clothes and take off your shoes.

And you can meditate in many different places wearing any type of clothing or no clothing at all. You can meditate while being a passenger in a car, bus, train, or plane.

You can meditate sitting or lying on the beach (perhaps your anchor would be the sound of the surf). You can meditate in an airport—some have small chapels or meditation rooms, or you can meditate right in the waiting area before boarding a plane.

⁂

Why do I sometimes feel like I am falling asleep when I meditate?

Feeling sleepy and/or falling asleep during the practice of meditation is very common. This probably means that you are in genuine need of some sleep. When you meditate, you tend to relax the body and mind. When you relax, you are more likely to receive clear signals from the body of what it actually needs. So, if during meditation you are feeling like you need to sleep, then you probably need some sleep. At that point, feel free to lie down and sleep and then wake up and meditate. Meditation is not about fighting sleep. If you have time to meditate, you have time for a quick nap.

⁂ ⁂ ⁂

Will I tend to stay on my anchor longer the more often I practice meditation?

Over time and on average, you will probably tend to stay on your anchor longer in between wanderings of the mind. You will probably also stay on your anchor longer overall during the course of the meditation the more often that you meditate. However, you may meditate for years and years and then sit down one day, and find your mind is wandering all over the place. The secret to getting the benefits of meditation is to relax about how skilled you are at staying on your anchor each time you meditate. Everyone's mind wanders to one degree or another.

⁂ ⁂ ⁂

What if during the meditation I am having thoughts that are really interesting or that I do not want to forget?

Often during meditation you may start to have thoughts that are very interesting or might be useful (for example, thoughts that might be useful for work). When this happens, you have a choice.

You can choose to notice that you are having these thoughts and then come back to your anchor, or you can choose to focus on the thoughts and end your meditation for the moment.

Do what you choose to do. Just realize that once you decide to focus on your thoughts, then you are not meditating. You may be doing something useful, such as contemplating or strategic planning or whatever, but you are not meditating. You are not going to be cultivating the benefits of meditation in that moment.

If after you notice this type of interesting thought, you choose to come back to your anchor and continue your meditation you may want to say the following to yourself, "This is a really interesting thought and may be useful. But right now I am meditating so I am going to come back to my anchor. I am going to trust that when I need to have this thought again, I will have it at the right time. I trust that this will happen so I am going back to my anchor—back to my meditation."

You will probably notice if you do this that most of the seemingly useful thoughts that occur during meditation are not lost forever if you choose not to focus on them, and that they will come back up to the conscious mind when you need them. Developing this trust in yourself and in the processes of your mind takes time and is another potential benefit of meditation.

A way to deal with this situation when you first start to meditate and you have not yet developed this trust is to keep a pad and pen next to you while you meditate. If a thought comes into your mind that you think is important and that you are afraid you might forget after the meditation, you can open your eyes, write the thought down (for example, "Call Mom after meditating"), and then go back to your meditation.

Is counting sheep meditating?

Yes, if you do it following the guidelines of meditation. You begin counting sheep, that is your anchor. When you notice that you are not counting sheep, you come back to counting sheep without worrying that for some moments you were thinking about something else.

Some people do not count sheep as a method of falling asleep because they know that they can not stay focused on the sheep, so they think it won't work. This is a major fallacy of counting sheep and a major fallacy of meditation. No one can stay focused on the sheep, just as no one can stay focused on his or her anchor in meditation.

You do not have to stay focused on your anchor. You are not trying to quiet the mind. You are not trying to do anything. Simply focus on the process and you will get the benefits of meditation.

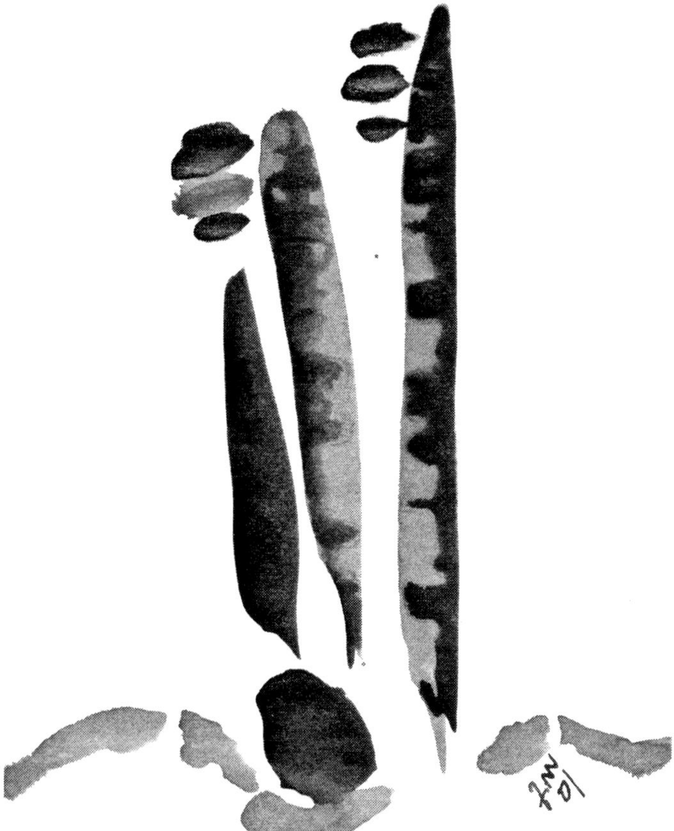

Conclusion

As you practice meditation, you will gain the benefits of relaxation, awareness, stress reduction, improved decision making, and an increased appreciation for life. For some people, these benefits may not be enough to motivate them to meditate.

Some people see these benefits as helping only themselves and think that it is a selfish act to spend time in meditation. They think they are too busy with family and work responsibilities to possibly spend a few minutes sitting with their eyes closed doing nothing when the only possible benefits seem to be for themselves.

This, however, is a narrow perspective. In fact, you are very directly helping those around you and in the world when you meditate. If you are more relaxed and accepting, have less stress, make better decisions, and have an increased appreciation for life, you are more likely to show more love and respect for people and animals and the world. Self growth and development are not selfish acts.

We all must take care of our own health and well being, through practices such as meditation, so that we can make our contribution to the world from a place of strength and peacefulness.

⁂ ⁂ ⁂

Meditation for Stress Reduction Workshops

Gary Halperin teaches the Feel Better Now Meditation technique privately and to corporate, civic, and governmental groups.

※ ※ ※

To arrange a workshop, send an email to:

garyhalperin@yahoo.com

Or visit:

www.feelbetternowyoga.com

About the art

Born in Canada, Frank Minogue now resides in Austin, Texas. His art ranges from the pen and ink washes highlighted here to paintings and metal sculptures. An author in his own right, Frank's children's book, *Little Horse* has been recently released.

⁂ ⁂ ⁂

Index